SIP YOUR WAY TO VITALITY

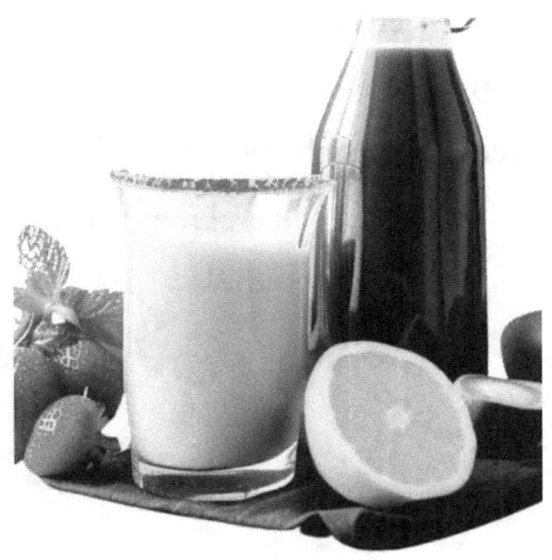

A Beginner's Guide to Juicing for Wellness and Health

Jessica L. Michael

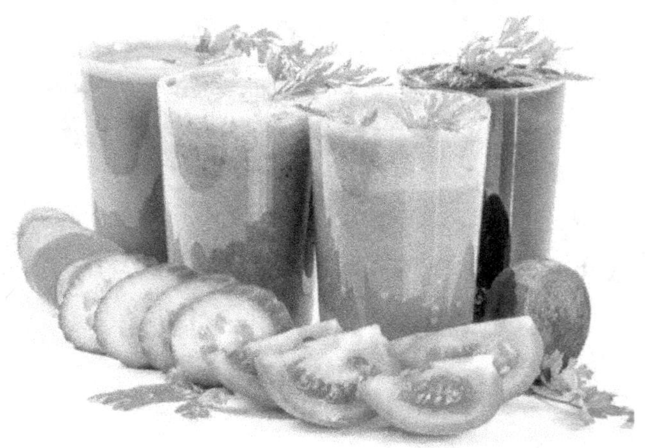

TABLE OF CONTENT

INTRODUCING

I had always been interested in healthy eating and living an active lifestyle. However, despite my best efforts, I often found myself struggling to maintain a balanced diet and stay motivated. That was until I discovered that juicing was another healthy way for general well-being.

At first, I was hesitant to try juicing. I had always been a bit intimidated by the thought of making my own juices and worried that I might not like the taste. But as I read and did some research, I felt more and more inspired to give it a try.

I purchased a juicer and began experimenting different recipes. I was pleasantly surprised by how easy it was to make delicious and nutritious juices and smoothies. I loved the variety of recipes, from detoxifying juices to energizing smoothies.

As I continued to incorporate juicing into my daily routine, I noticed a significant improvement in my overall health and well-being. I had more energy, felt more focused, and even slept better at night. My skin looked clearer and more radiant, and I no longer felt bloated or sluggish after meals.

This made me so excited by the positive changes have experienced within a short period of time with juicing I have discovered a new passion for healthy living and found a means to motivate others to follow suit. Am so excited to explore the world of juicing and sharing my discoveries with others.

The Benefits of Juicing for Health and Wellness

In recent years, there has been a surge in the popularity of juicing, and this trend is well-justified. The process of extracting the juice from fruits and vegetables allows us to consume a concentrated dose of vitamins, minerals, and antioxidants that are essential for our health and well-being.

One of the primary benefits of juicing is that it can help to detoxify the body. By consuming fresh, nutrient-rich juice, we can help to flush out toxins and other harmful substances from our system, leaving us feeling more energized and rejuvenated.

Juicing can also be an effective tool for weight loss. By replacing high-calorie, processed foods with fresh juice, we can reduce our overall calorie intake while still providing our bodies with the nutrients they need to function properly.

In addition, juicing can help to fight the signs of aging. The antioxidants and other compounds found in fruits and vegetables can help to protect our cells from damage caused by free radicals, which can lead to premature aging and disease.

Overall, the benefits of juicing for health and wellness are numerous.

1. **Increased hydration:** Juicing is an excellent way to increase your daily water intake. The high water content of fruits and vegetables helps to keep your body hydrated, which is essential for optimal health.

2. **Improved digestion:** Juicing can help to improve digestion by breaking down food more easily and reducing the workload of the digestive system. This can lead to better absorption of nutrients and less digestive discomfort.

3. **Better skin health:** The antioxidants and other nutrients found in fruits and vegetables can help to improve skin health, reducing the signs of aging and promoting a clear, glowing complexion.

4. **Increased mental clarity:** The vitamins, minerals, and other nutrients found in fresh juice can help to improve cognitive function, including memory, focus, and concentration.

5. **Reduced inflammation:** Juicing can help to reduce inflammation throughout the body, which is associated with a wide range of health problems, including chronic pain, autoimmune disorders, and even cancer.

Ways this book can aid you in commencing your juicing journey?

If you're interested in incorporating juicing into your lifestyle but aren't sure where to start, **"Sip your way to vitality: A beginner's Guide to juicing for wellness and health "** can be a valuable resource. Here are a few ways this book can help you get started with juicing:

1. **Beginner-friendly recipes:** The book is filled with easy-to-follow recipes that are perfect for beginners. You'll find a wide variety of recipes for juices, smoothies, and other healthy drinks that are packed with vitamins, minerals, and other nutrients.

2. **Nutritional information:** Each recipe in the book comes with detailed nutritional information, so you can be sure you're getting the right balance of nutrients for your body's needs.

3. **Tips and tricks:** The book also includes tips and tricks for getting the most out of your juicing experience. You'll learn about the best types of produce to use, how to store your juice to keep it fresh, and other helpful hints.

4. **Customizable recipes:** Many of the recipes in the book can be customized to suit your taste preferences or dietary needs. Whether you're looking for a low-sugar option or want to add more protein to your drinks, the book provides guidance on how to modify recipes to meet your needs.

Overall, **"Sip your way to vitality"** is a comprehensive guide that can help you get started with juicing and make the most of this powerful health practice.

CHAPTER ONE

THE BASICS OF JUICING

WHAT IS JUICING?

Juicing involves separating the juice or liquid from fruits and vegetables, while discarding the fiber and pulp. The resulting juice is a concentrated source of vitamins, minerals, and other nutrients that are essential for good health.

There are many different ways to juice, from using a simple handheld juicer to a high-powered juicing machine. Some people also choose to blend their fruits and vegetables into smoothies, which retain more of the fiber and other plant materials.

Juicing has become increasingly popular in recent years as a way to improve health and well-being. Proponents of juicing believe that it can help to detoxify the body, improve digestion, boost energy levels, and even reduce the risk of chronic disease.

However, it's important to note that juicing should not be seen as a replacement for whole fruits and vegetables in the diet. While juicing can be a great way to consume a concentrated dose of nutrients, it's still important to eat a varied diet that includes a range of whole, plant-based foods for optimal health.

The Different Types of Juicers

There are several different types of juicers on the market, each with its own unique features and benefits. The following are the most prevalent kinds of juicers:

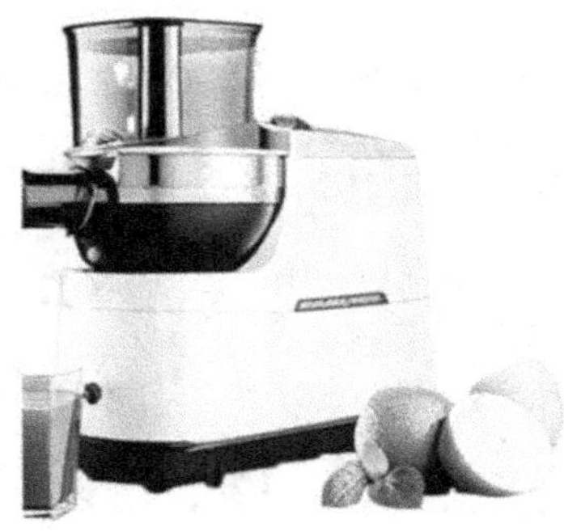

1. **Centrifugal juicers:** These juicers work by grinding fruits and vegetables into a pulp and then spinning the pulp at a high speed to separate the juice from the solids. They are generally fast and easy to use, but may not be as effective at juicing leafy greens or producing a high yield of juice.

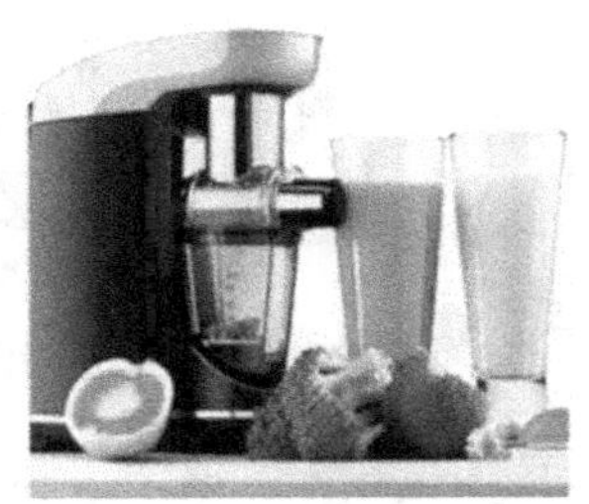

2. **Masticating juicers:** Also known as slow juicers, masticating juicers use a slow, grinding motion to extract juice from fruits and vegetables. They are generally more efficient at extracting juice and can handle a wider range of produce than centrifugal juicers, but they are also more expensive and slower to operate.

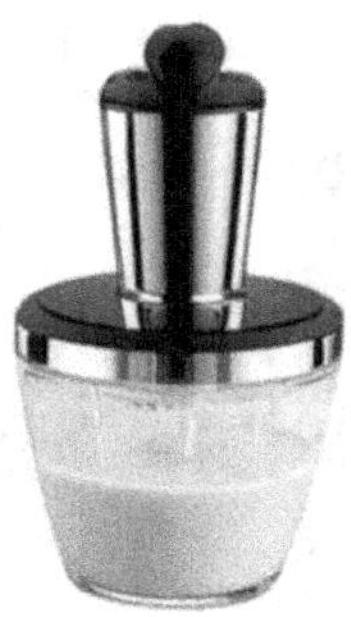 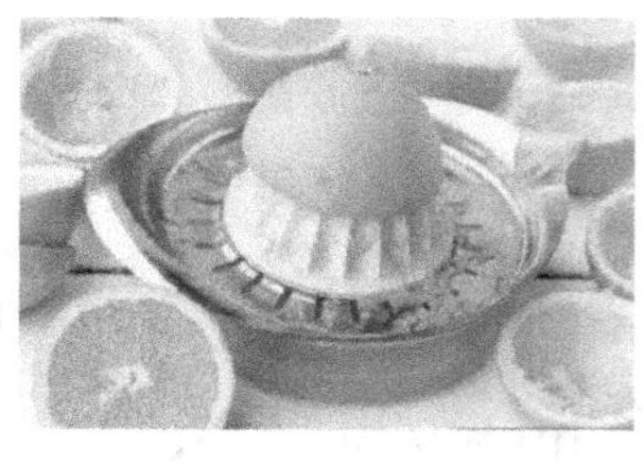

3. **Citrus juicers:** As the name suggests, citrus juicers are designed specifically for juicing citrus fruits such as oranges, lemons, and grapefruits. They can be manual or electric and are generally affordable and easy to use.

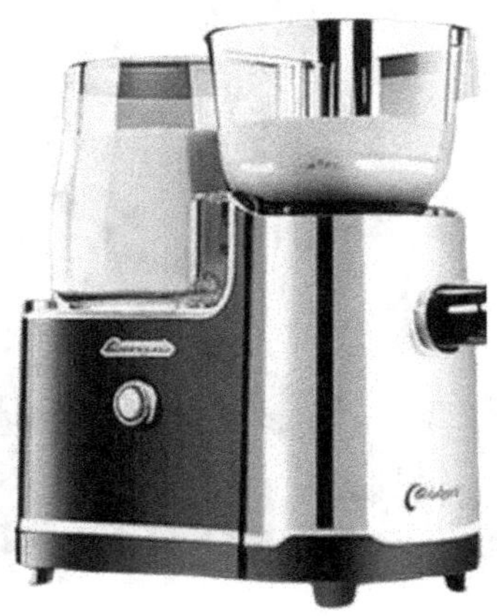

4. **Twin-gear juicers:** These juicers use two interlocking gears to crush fruits and vegetables and extract the juice. They are generally considered to be the most efficient type of juicer and are capable of producing a high yield of juice from even the toughest produce; however, these types of juicers are also the costliest and most challenging to clean.

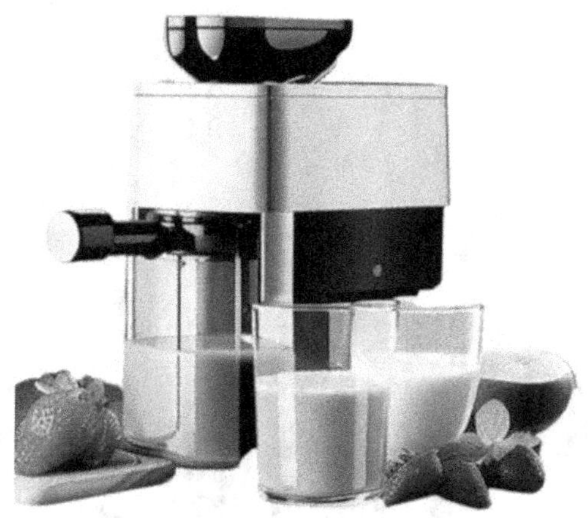

5. **Hydraulic press juicers:** These juicers use a hydraulic press to extract juice from fruits and vegetables. They are generally the most expensive type of juicer but also produce the highest quality juice with the most nutrients intact.

When choosing a juicer, it's important to consider your budget, the types of produce you plan to juice, and your personal preferences for ease of use and cleaning.

Choosing the Right Juicer for You

When it comes to choosing the right juicer for you, there are several factors to consider. Consider the following important factors:

1. **Type of produce**: Consider the types of fruits and vegetables you plan to juice most often. If you'll be juicing a lot of leafy greens, a masticating juicer may be a better choice than a centrifugal juicer.

2. **Budget:** Juicers can range in price from under $50 to over $1,000. Think about your budget and prioritize the features that matter to you.

3. **Ease of use:** Some juicers are easier to use than others, with features like wide feed chutes and self-cleaning mechanisms. If you want to be able to make juice quickly and easily, look for a juicer with user-friendly features.

4. **Yield and efficiency:** Different juicers can produce different amounts of juice from the same amount of produce. Consider how important it is to you to get the most juice possible from your fruits and vegetables.

5. **Maintenance and cleaning:** Juicers can be a pain to clean, so consider how much time and effort you're willing to put into cleaning your juicer. Some models are easier to clean than others, with dishwasher-safe parts and simple disassembly.

In the end, the most suitable juicer for you will be based on your specific requirements and personal choices. Consider your budget, the types of produce you'll be juicing, and your desired level of ease of use and maintenance when making your decision.

Tips for Juicing Success

Juicing can be a great way to incorporate more fruits and vegetables into your diet, but it can also be a bit intimidating if you're new to it. Here are some tips for juicing success:

1. **Choose the right produce:** Make sure to choose fresh, ripe fruits and vegetables for juicing. This will ensure that you get the most flavor and nutrients from your juice.

2. **Experiment with different combinations:** Don't be afraid to try new combinations of fruits and vegetables to find what you like best. You may be surprised at how well certain flavors and textures work together.

3. **Prep your produce:** Wash your produce thoroughly and cut it into small pieces that will fit easily into your juicer. This will help

ensure that your juicer operates smoothly and efficiently.

4. **Drink your juice immediately:** Fresh juice is best consumed immediately after juicing, as it can lose nutrients and flavor quickly. If you are unable to consume your juice immediately, keep it in a sealed container in the refrigerator for a maximum of 24 hours.

5. **Clean your juicer thoroughly:** Juicers can be difficult to clean, but it's important to do so after each use to prevent bacteria growth and ensure that your juicer operates properly. Follow the manufacturer's instructions for cleaning your juicer, and be sure to take it apart completely to clean all parts.

6. **Don't overdo it:** While juicing can be a healthy addition to your diet, it's important not to overdo it. Drinking too much juice can lead to an excessive intake of sugar and

calories, which can be counterproductive to your health goals.

By following these tips, you can set yourself up for success when it comes to juicing. Remember to have fun and experiment with different flavors and combinations to find what works best for you.

Difference between Juicing and Blending

Juicing and blending are both popular ways to incorporate more fruits and vegetables into your diet, but they are different processes with different outcomes.

Juicing involves extracting the liquid from fruits and vegetables, leaving behind the pulp and fiber. This results in a nutrient-dense juice that is easy to digest and absorb. Juicing can be a great way to quickly and easily consume a large amount of fruits and vegetables, but it can also be relatively low in fiber.

Blending, on the other hand, involves blending whole fruits and vegetables into a thick, smooth consistency. This includes the pulp and fiber, which can help slow down the absorption of sugar and keep you feeling full. Blending can be a great way to incorporate more fiber into your diet, but it can also be more time-consuming and require a more powerful blender.

In summary, the main differences between juicing and blending are that juicing extracts the liquid from fruits and vegetables while leaving behind the fiber, while blending incorporates the whole fruit or vegetable, including the fiber. Both methods have their benefits and drawbacks, and the choice between juicing and blending ultimately depends on your individual preferences and goals.

The Different Health Benefit of Juicing and Blending

Juicing and blending both have their unique health benefits, as well as some similarities. Here are some of the key differences in the health benefits of juicing vs. blending:

Juicing:

1. **Increased nutrient absorption:** Juicing allows your body to quickly and easily absorb a concentrated amount of nutrients from fruits and vegetables, without the added fiber.

2. **Boosts immunity:** Juicing can help boost your immune system by providing a high dose of antioxidants, vitamins, and minerals.

3. **Detoxification:** Juicing is often used as part of a detox or cleanse, as it can help flush toxins from the body and improve digestion.

4. **Lowers inflammation:** Some research suggests that juicing can help lower inflammation in the body, which is linked to many chronic diseases.

Blending:

1. **Fiber intake:** Blending incorporates the whole fruit or vegetable, including the fiber, which can help keep you feeling full and regulate blood sugar levels.

2. **Improved digestion:** The fiber in blended fruits and vegetables can help improve digestion and prevent constipation.

3. **Satiety:** Blending can help keep you feeling full for longer periods of time, which can help with weight management.

4. **Maintains nutrient content:** Blending doesn't expose fruits and vegetables to as much heat and air as juicing, so the nutrients are more likely to be preserved.

In summary, while both juicing and blending can be beneficial to your health, they each have their unique advantages. Juicing provides a concentrated dose of nutrients and can aid in detoxification, while blending incorporates fiber and can help with digestion and satiety.

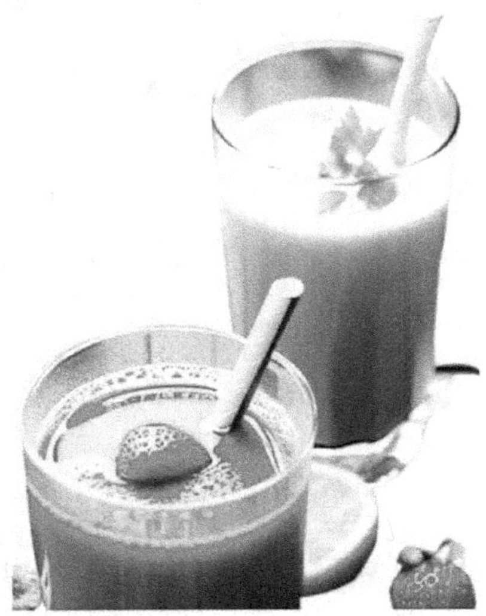

CHAPTER TWO

GETTING STARTED WITH JUICING

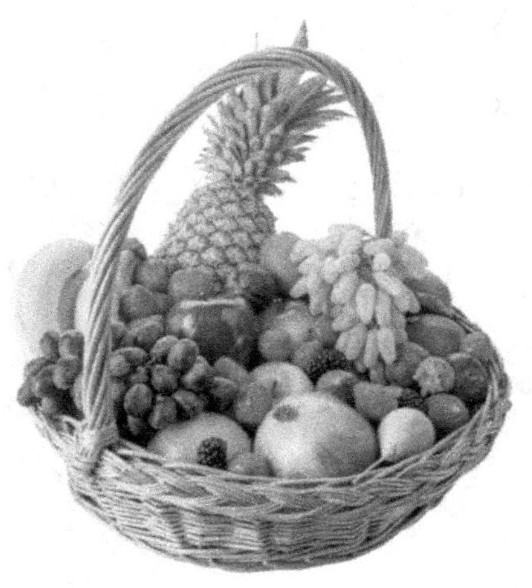

THE BEST FRUITS AND VEGETABLES FOR JUICING

When it comes to juicing, some fruits and vegetables are better suited than others due to their flavor, nutrient content, and juiciness. Here are some of the best fruits and vegetables for juicing:

1. **Leafy greens:** Kale, spinach, Swiss chard, and collard greens are all excellent sources of vitamins and minerals and are highly nutritious when juiced.

2. **Citrus fruits:** Oranges, lemons, limes, and grapefruits are all rich in vitamin C and can add a refreshing tang to your juice.

3. **Carrots:** Carrots are sweet and highly nutritious, providing a good source of vitamin A, potassium, and fiber.

4. **Beets:** Beets are rich in antioxidants and can help support liver function and detoxification.

5. **Apples:** Apples are naturally sweet and can add a pleasant flavor to your juice, while also providing a good source of vitamin C and fiber.

6. **Ginger:** Adding fresh ginger to your juice can provide a spicy kick while also offering

anti-inflammatory and digestion-boosting benefits.

7. **Cucumbers:** Cucumbers are refreshing and hydrating, making them a great addition to your juice.

8. **Pineapple:** Pineapple contains an enzyme called bromelain, which can help aid in digestion and reduce inflammation.

9. **Celery:** Celery is hydrating and contains antioxidants and anti-inflammatory compounds that can help support overall health.

10. **Berries:** Blueberries, strawberries, raspberries, and blackberries are all packed with antioxidants and can add a delicious sweetness to your juice.

11. **Parsley:** Parsley is a great source of vitamin C and can add a fresh, herbaceous flavor to your juice.

12. **Watermelon:** Watermelon is high in vitamin C and contains the amino acid citrulline, which can help improve circulation and lower blood pressure.

13. **Pears:** Pears are naturally sweet and can add a subtle flavor to your juice, while also providing a good source of fiber.

14. **Broccoli:** Broccoli is a cruciferous vegetable that is high in vitamin C and other antioxidants, and can help support detoxification and reduce inflammation.

15. **Turmeric:** Adding fresh turmeric to your juice can provide anti-inflammatory and antioxidant benefits, and add a warm, earthy flavor.

When juicing, it's important to aim for a variety of fruits and vegetables to ensure you're getting a wide range of nutrients. Additionally, it's important to choose organic produce whenever possible to reduce exposure to pesticides and other harmful chemicals.

Remember to experiment with different combinations of fruits and vegetables to find your perfect juice blend, and don't be afraid to add herbs and spices to enhance the flavor and health benefits of your juice.

The Importance of Organic Produce

When it comes to juicing, choosing organic produce can be an important factor in ensuring you're getting the most nutrient-dense and health-promoting juice possible. Here are some reasons why organic produce is important:

1. **Fewer pesticides:** Conventionally grown produce is often sprayed with pesticides and herbicides to ward off pests and weeds. These

chemicals can be harmful to human health, and choosing organic produce reduces exposure to these toxins.

2. **More nutrients:** Organic produce is often grown in nutrient-rich soil without the use of synthetic fertilizers, resulting in produce that is higher in vitamins, minerals, and other beneficial compounds.

3. **Better for the environment:** Organic farming practices prioritize soil health, biodiversity, and sustainability, making it a more eco-friendly choice.

4. **Supporting small farmers:** Buying organic produce from local farmers can help support small-scale agriculture and promote local food systems.

While organic produce can be more expensive, it's important to prioritize buying organic for the fruits and vegetables that are most heavily sprayed with pesticides, such as strawberries, spinach, and apples. When shopping for organic produce, look for the USDA Organic label to ensure that the produce meets strict organic standards.

How to Prepare Your Produce for Juicing

Properly preparing your produce is an important step in getting the most out of your juicing experience. Here are some tips for preparing your fruits and vegetables for juicing:

1. **Wash your produce:** Rinse your fruits and vegetables thoroughly with cool water to remove any dirt or debris. You can also use a produce wash to help remove any residue.

2. **Cut your produce into manageable pieces:** Depending on the size of your juicer, you may need to cut larger fruits and vegetables

into smaller pieces. For example, you may need to cut an apple into quarters or chop up a head of kale into smaller pieces.

3. **Remove any inedible parts:** Be sure to remove any parts of the produce that are not edible, such as stems or seeds. Some produce, like citrus fruits, may need to have the peel removed.

4. **Chill your produce:** To help keep your juice cool and fresh, you can store your produce in the refrigerator or freezer before juicing.

5. **Juice immediately:** For the most nutritious juice, it's best to juice your produce immediately after preparing it. However, if you need to store your juice for later, be sure to store it in an airtight container in the refrigerator and consume it within 24-48 hours.

By following these tips, you can ensure that your produce is properly prepared and ready to be juiced into a delicious and nutritious beverage.

Basic Juicing Recipes to Get You Started

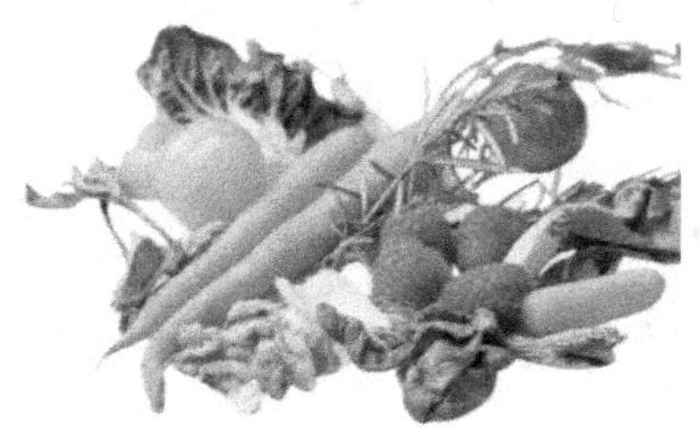

Below are some simple juicing recipes to help you begin:

1.   **Green Juice:**

   - 2 cups spinach
   - 1 cucumber
   - 1 apple
   - 1/2 lemon

Green Juice: This recipe is packed with nutrients like vitamin C, iron, and calcium from the spinach, and hydration from the cucumber. The apple and lemon provide a touch of sweetness and tartness, respectively, while adding additional vitamins and antioxidants.

2.   Carrot-Apple Juice:

- 3-4 carrots
- 2 apples
- 1/2 inch piece of ginger

Carrot-Apple Juice: This recipe is high in vitamin A from the carrots, as well as vitamin C and fiber from the apples. The ginger adds a spicy kick and also has anti-inflammatory properties.

3.   Beet-Orange Juice:

- 1 beet
- 2 oranges
- 1 carrot

Beet-Orange Juice: This recipe is high in vitamin C and folate from the oranges, while the beet provides a boost of antioxidants and can help to improve blood flow and lower blood pressure.

4.   Pineapple-Mint Juice:

- 1/4 pineapple
- 1/2 cucumber
- 1/4 cup mint leaves

Pineapple-Mint Juice: This recipe is a refreshing way to hydrate, with the pineapple providing vitamin C and bromelain, an enzyme that can aid in digestion. The cucumber adds hydration, while the mint provides a burst of flavor and can help to soothe digestion.

5.   Strawberry-Kiwi Juice:

- 1 cup strawberries
- 2 kiwis
- 1/2 lime

Strawberry-Kiwi Juice: This recipe is high in vitamin C from the strawberries and kiwis, while the lime provides additional vitamin C and antioxidants. The combination of sweet and tart flavors makes for a refreshing and delicious juice.

To make these juices, simply run the ingredients through your juicer and enjoy. You can also experiment with different combinations of fruits and vegetables to create your own unique juicing recipes. Remember to choose organic produce whenever possible and to properly prepare your produce before juicing for optimal flavor and nutrition.

These basic juicing recipes provide a variety of nutrients, including vitamins, minerals, and antioxidants, that can help to support overall health and wellness. Remember to use fresh, organic produce whenever possible for the best flavor and nutritional benefits.

CHAPTER THREE

JUICING FOR HEALTH AND WELLNESS

DETOXIFICATION: WHY AND HOW TO DO IT

Detoxification involves the elimination of harmful toxins from the body. It is important to detoxify your body regularly as toxins can build up over time and cause damage to your organs, immune system, and overall health. Here are some reasons why and how to do it:

1. **Remove Toxins:** Detoxifying your body can help remove harmful toxins that accumulate from the air you breathe, the foods you eat, and the products you use. This can help

reduce the risk of chronic diseases and improve overall health.

2.   **Boost Immunity:** A healthy body is better equipped to fight off illness and disease. Detoxification can help boost your immune system by removing toxins and supporting the body's natural defense mechanisms.

3.   **Improve Digestion:** Detoxification can improve digestion by removing harmful toxins that can cause inflammation and irritation in the digestive tract. Detoxification can aid in alleviating digestive problems such as bloating and gas by eliminating harmful toxins from the body.

4.   **Increase Energy:** Detoxification can help increase energy levels by removing toxins that can cause fatigue and sluggishness. Incorporating juicing into your daily routine

can aid in improving your alertness and focus.

To detoxify your body, there are many approaches you can take, such as:

1. Eating a healthy, whole-foods-based diet that is rich in fruits, vegetables, and fiber.

2. Staying hydrated by drinking plenty of water and herbal teas.

3. Engaging in regular exercise to promote sweating and release toxins through the skin.

4. Avoiding alcohol, caffeine, and processed foods that can be high in toxins.

5. Trying various detoxification methods such as juice fasting, sauna sessions, or colon cleansing, under the guidance of a healthcare professional.

Remember, it is important to consult with your healthcare provider before beginning any detoxification program to ensure that it is safe and effective for you.

Recipes for Detoxification Juices and Smoothies and nutritional values

Detoxification juices and smoothies can be a great way to support your body's natural cleansing processes. Below are some juicing recipes that you can try out:

1.   Green Detox Juice:

Ingredients
- 2 cups kale
- 2 cups spinach
- 1 green apple
- 1 lemon, juiced
- 1 inch fresh ginger root
- 1 cup water

Preparation: Wash all ingredients thoroughly

Combine all the ingredients in a juicer and extract the juice.

Green Detox Juice Nutritional value

- Calories: 97
- Protein: 5g
- Fat: 1g
- Carbohydrates: 25g
- Fiber: 6g
- Sugar: 14g
- Vitamin A: 601% DV
- Vitamin C: 340% DV
- Calcium: 15% DV
- Iron: 3% DV

2.   **Berry Detox Smoothie:**

Ingredients

- 1 cup of assorted berries, which may include blueberries, raspberries, and strawberries.
- 1 banana
- 1 cup unsweetened almond milk
- 1 tablespoon chia seeds

- 1 teaspoon honey (optional)

Preparation: Blend all ingredients together until smooth. Serve immediately.

Berry Detox Smoothie nutritional value

- Calories: 240
- Protein: 4g
- Fat: 9g
- Carbohydrates: 39g
- Fiber: 9g
- Sugar: 22g
- Vitamin A: 5% DV
- Vitamin C: 119% DV
- Calcium: 37% DV
- Iron: 2% DV

3.   Carrot and Ginger Detox Juice:

Ingredients

- 4 carrots
- 1 inch fresh ginger root
- 1 apple
- 1 lemon, juiced
- 1 cup water

Preparation: Wash all ingredients thoroughly

Combine all the ingredients in a juicer and extract the juice.

Carrot and Ginger Detox Juice nutritional value

- Calories: 130
- Protein: 4g
- Fat: 1g
- Carbohydrates: 30g
- Fiber: 6g
- Sugar: 16g
- Vitamin A: 874% DV
- Vitamin C: 117% DV
- Calcium: 12% DV
- Iron: 3% DV

4. Green Smoothie:

Ingredients

- 1 cup spinach
- 1 banana
- 1 kiwi
- 1/2 cup pineapple
- 1/2 cup unsweetened almond milk

Preparation: Blend all ingredients together until smooth. Serve immediately.

Green Smoothie nutritional value

- Calories: 184
- Protein: 4g
- Fat: 2g
- Carbohydrates: 43g
- Fiber: 8g
- Sugar: 23g
- Vitamin A: 95% DV
- Vitamin C: 172% DV
- Calcium: 21% DV
- Iron: 2% DV

5.   **Beet and Carrot Detox Juice:**

Ingredients

- 2 beets
- 2 carrots
- 1 lemon, juiced
- 1 inch fresh ginger root
- 1 cup water

Preparation: Wash all ingredients thoroughly

Combine all the ingredients in a juicer and extract the juice.

Beet and Carrot Detox Juice nutritional value

- Calories: 140
- Protein: 4g
- Fat: 1g
- Carbohydrates: 35g
- Fiber: 8g
- Sugar: 21g
- Vitamin A: 609% DV
- Vitamin C: 155% DV
- Calcium: 8% DV
- Iron: 3% DV

6.   Avocado Detox Smoothie:

Ingredients

- 1 avocado
- 1/2 cucumber
- 1/2 lime, juiced
- 1/2 cup coconut water
- 1/2 cup unsweetened almond milk

Preparation: Blend all ingredients together until smooth. Serve immediately.

Avocado Detox Smoothie nutritional value

- Calories: 278
- Protein: 5g
- Fat: 19g
- Carbohydrates: 25g
- Fiber: 11g
- Sugar: 8g
- Vitamin A: 15% DV
- Vitamin C: 23% DV
- Calcium: 10% DV
- Iron: 5% DV

Please note that these nutritional values may vary depending on the specific brands and amounts of ingredients used. Remember to consult with your healthcare provider before beginning any detoxification program to ensure that it is safe and effective for you. Additionally, these recipes can be incorporated into a healthy diet but should not be used as a substitute for meals or a balanced diet.

Weight Loss: How Juicing Can Help

Juicing can be a helpful tool for weight loss because it allows you to consume more fruits and vegetables in a concentrated form. Here are some ways juicing can aid in weight loss:

1. **Low in calories:** Juices are typically low in calories and can help you reduce your overall calorie intake. By substituting a juice for a higher calorie meal or snack, you can reduce your daily calorie intake and potentially lose weight.

2. **High in fiber:** Some juices, especially those made with fruits and vegetables high in fiber, can help you feel fuller for longer. This can

aid in curbing your hunger and avoiding excessive consumption.

3. **Boosts metabolism:** Certain fruits and vegetables, such as ginger and grapefruit, can help boost metabolism and promote weight loss.

4. **Provides nutrients:** Juices can be a great way to get essential nutrients, such as vitamins and minerals, that your body needs for optimal health. When your body is properly nourished, it can be easier to lose weight.

5. **Hydrates the body:** Juices are also a great source of hydration, which is important for weight loss. When you are properly hydrated, your body can function more efficiently and burn more calories.

Overall, incorporating juicing into a healthy weight loss plan can be a great way to boost your nutrient intake, reduce your calorie intake, and promote weight loss.

Recipes for Weight Loss Juices and Smoothies and Preparation Method and Their Nutritional Value

Here are some recipes for weight loss juices and smoothies, along with their preparation method and nutritional value:

1.   Green Apple and Kale Juice:

Ingredients:
- 2 green apples
- 2 cups kale
- 1 cucumber
- 1/2 lemon
- 1 inch piece of ginger

Preparation:

- Wash all ingredients thoroughly
- Cut apples and cucumber into pieces
- Combine all the ingredients in a juicer and extract the juice.
- Serve immediately

Nutritional Value:
- Calories: 170
- Carbohydrates: 44g
- Protein: 6g
- Fat: 1g
- Fiber: 13g
- Sugar: 28g

2.　　Strawberry and Banana Smoothie:

Ingredients:
- 1 banana
- 1 cup strawberries
- 1/2 cup almond milk
- 1 tbsp honey

Preparation:
- Wash all ingredients thoroughly
- Cut banana and strawberries into pieces
- Combine all ingredients in a blender and blend until a smooth consistency is achieved."
- Serve immediately

Nutritional Value:
- Calories: 170
- Carbohydrates: 39g
- Protein: 3g
- Fat: 2g
- Fiber: 6g
- Sugar: 25g

3.   Beetroot and Carrot Juice:

Ingredients:
- 1 medium-sized beetroot
- 2 large carrots
- 1/2 lemon

Preparation:
- Wash all ingredients thoroughly
- Peel the beetroot and carrots
- Cut into pieces
- Combine all the ingredients in a juicer and extract the juice.
- Serve immediately

Nutritional Value:
- Calories: 110
- Carbohydrates: 26g
- Protein: 3g
- Fat: 1g
- Fiber: 8g
- Sugar: 18g

4. Green Apple and Spinach Smoothie:

Ingredients

- Ingredients: 1 green apple
- 2 cups of spinach
- 1 banana
- 1/2 cup of almond milk
- 1 teaspoon of honey

Preparation: Blend all ingredients until smooth

Nutritional Value: 173 calories, 5g protein, 42g carbohydrates, 3g fat, 8g fiber

5. Pineapple and Ginger Juice:

Ingredients:

- 2 cups of pineapple
- 1 inch piece of ginger
- 1 cucumber
- 1 lemon

Preparation:

- Juice all ingredients together

Nutritional Value: 119 calories, 3g protein, 29g carbohydrates, 1g fat, 2g fiber

These juices and smoothies can be a healthy addition to a weight loss plan. It's important to remember that weight loss is not just about juicing, but rather a combination of healthy eating habits and physical activity.

Anti-Aging: How Juicing Can Help You Look and Feel Younger

Juicing is not only beneficial for detoxification and weight loss, but it can also help slow down the aging process. As we age, our body's ability to absorb nutrients declines, but by incorporating certain fruits and vegetables into our diet through juicing, we can provide our body with the necessary vitamins and minerals to keep us looking and feeling young.

In this section, we will explore the different types of fruits and vegetables that are known for their anti-aging properties and provide recipes for juices and smoothies that can help you achieve a more youthful complexion and boost your energy levels.

Some of the best fruits and vegetables for anti-aging include **berries, leafy greens, avocado, cucumber, and carrots.** By juicing these ingredients together, we can create a potent blend of antioxidants, vitamins, and minerals that can help improve our skin's texture, prevent wrinkles, and promote overall health.

Anti-aging juice and smoothie recipes along with their preparation method and nutritional value:

1.   Green Machine Juice:

Ingredients:
  *   2 cups of spinach

- 1 green apple
- 1 cucumber
- 1 lemon
- 1 inch of ginger

Preparation: Wash and chop all the ingredients, then put them through a juicer. Serve over ice.

Nutritional Value: This juice is packed with Vitamin C, Vitamin A, iron, and antioxidants, which help to reduce inflammation and promote healthy aging.

2. Avocado-Berry Smoothie:

Ingredients:
- 1/2 avocado
- 1 cup of mixed berries
- 1 banana
- 1 cup of almond milk
- 1 tsp of honey

Preparation: Combine all ingredients in a blender and blend until smooth. Add ice if desired.

Nutritional Value: This smoothie is high in healthy fats, fiber, Vitamin C, and antioxidants, which can help improve skin elasticity and promote a youthful glow.

3. **Carrot-Orange Juice:**

Ingredients:

- 3 carrots
- 1 orange
- 1/2 lemon

Preparation: Wash and peel the carrots, then juice them along with the orange and lemon. Serve over ice.

Nutritional Value: This juice is high in Vitamin A, Vitamin C, and antioxidants, which can help protect against damage from free radicals and promote healthy skin.

4.   Kale-Pineapple Smoothie:

Ingredients:

- 2 cups of kale
- 1 cup of pineapple
- 1 banana
- 1/2 cup of coconut water
- 1 tbsp of chia seeds

Preparation: Combine all ingredients in a blender and blend until smooth. Add ice if desired.

Nutritional Value: This smoothie is packed with antioxidants, fiber, and Vitamin C, which can help reduce

inflammation and improve skin
texture.

5.   **Beet-Berry Juice:**

Ingredients:

- 1 beetroot
- 1 cup of mixed berries
- 1/2 lemon

Preparation: Wash and chop the beetroot, then juice it along with the berries and lemon. Serve over ice.

Nutritional Value: This juice is high in antioxidants, iron, and Vitamin C, which can help improve blood flow and promote healthy aging.

CHAPTER FOUR

JUICING FOR SPECIFIC HEALTH CONCERNS

BOOSTING YOUR IMMUNE SYSTEM: HOW JUICING CAN HELP

Juicing can help boost your immune system by providing your body with essential nutrients that are necessary for optimal health. When you juice fruits and vegetables, you get a concentrated dose of vitamins, minerals, and antioxidants that can help support your immune system and keep you healthy. Here are some tips for boosting your immune system with juicing:

1. **Choose fruits and vegetables that are high in vitamin C,** such as oranges, grapefruits, kiwis, strawberries, and bell peppers. Vitamin

C is an antioxidant that can help protect your cells from damage and boost your immune system.

2. **Add ginger to your juices and smoothies.** Ginger has anti-inflammatory properties that can help reduce inflammation in your body and improve your immune function.

3. Include leafy greens, such as spinach and kale, in your juices and smoothies. These greens are packed with vitamins and minerals that are essential for immune function.

4. **Add garlic to your juices and smoothies.** Garlic has antibacterial and antiviral properties that can help support your immune system and protect your body from infection.

5. **Use turmeric in your juices and smoothies.** Turmeric contains curcumin, a powerful antioxidant that can help reduce inflammation and improve immune function.

Recipes for immune-boosting juices and smoothies with preparation method and nutritional value:

1.   Citrus Immune Booster Juice:

Ingredients

- 2 oranges
- 1 grapefruit
- 1 lemon
- 1 inch piece of ginger

Preparation:

- Peel the citrus fruits and ginger, and juice them using a juicer. Serve immediately.

Nutritional value: 157 calories, 39g carbs, 4g protein, 1g fat, 7g fiber

2.   Green Immune Booster Smoothie:

Ingredients

1 cup spinach

- 1 cup kale
- 1 green apple
- 1/2 cucumber
- 1/2 lemon
- 1 inch piece of ginger

Preparation: Combine all the ingredients to a blender and blend until smooth. Serve immediately.

Nutritional value: 126 calories, 30g carbs, 3g protein, 1g fat, 7g fiber

3. Carrot Turmeric Immune Booster Juice:

Ingredients

- 4 carrots
- 1 orange
- 1 inch piece of ginger
- 1 tsp turmeric powder

Preparation:
- Peel the carrots and ginger, and juice them along with the orange using a juicer.

- Add the turmeric powder and stir well. Serve immediately.

Nutritional value: 163 calories, 40g carbs, 4g protein, 1g fat, 7g fiber

4. **Pineapple Ginger Immune Booster Smoothie:**

Ingredients

- 1 cup pineapple chunks
- 1 inch piece of ginger
- 1/2 cup coconut water
- 1/2 banana

Combine all the ingredients to a blender and blend until smooth. Serve immediately.

Nutritional value: 131 calories, 32g carbs, 2g protein, 1g fat, 4g fiber

5. **Beetroot Orange Immune Booster Juice:**

Ingredients

- •	1 beetroot
- •	1 orange
- •	1 inch piece of ginger

Preparation:
- • Peel the beetroot and ginger, and juice them along with the orange using a juicer. Serve immediately.

Nutritional value: 145 calories, 34g carbs, 4g protein, 1g fat, 9g fiber

Managing Stress: How Juicing Can Help

Juicing can be a helpful tool in managing stress by providing the body with essential nutrients and vitamins that help to combat the negative effects of stress. Here are some ways juicing can help with stress management:

1. **Provides a natural source of energy:** Juices made from fruits and vegetables can provide

a natural source of energy, helping to combat fatigue and sluggishness that can contribute to stress.

2. **Contains stress-reducing vitamins and minerals:** Certain vitamins and minerals found in fruits and vegetables, such as vitamin C, magnesium, and potassium, can help to reduce stress and promote relaxation.

3. **Can help with hydration:** Staying hydrated is essential for stress management, as dehydration can increase feelings of stress and anxiety. Juicing can help to increase hydration levels by providing a source of water and electrolytes.

4. **Offers a convenient way to consume fruits and vegetables:** Juicing provides a convenient way to consume a variety of fruits and vegetables, even for those who may not enjoy eating them whole. This can help to

ensure a balanced and nutrient-rich diet, which can contribute to overall stress reduction.

5. **May help to reduce inflammation**: Chronic inflammation has been linked to an increased risk of stress-related disorders such as depression and anxiety. Some fruits and vegetables contain anti-inflammatory compounds that can help to reduce inflammation in the body.

Overall, incorporating juicing into a stress management routine can be a helpful way to support overall health and wellness.

Recipes for Stress-Relief Juices and Smoothies with preparation method and nutritional value

1.   **Blueberry Lavender Smoothie**

Ingredients:

- 1 cup blueberries
- 1 frozen banana
- 1 cup almond milk
- 1 tablespoon honey
- 1 teaspoon dried lavender
- Ice (optional)

Preparation:

- Combine all ingredients to a blender and blend until smooth.

- Add ice if desired, serve and enjoy immediately.

Nutritional value: Calories: 275; Fat: 3.7g; Carbohydrates: 59.6g; Fiber: 7.4g; Protein: 4.4g

2.   Mango Ginger Juice

Ingredients:

- 2 ripe mangoes, peeled and chopped
- 1-inch piece of ginger, then peeled and grated.
- 1 lemon, juiced
- 1 tablespoon honey
- 1 cup water

Preparation:

- Combine all ingredients to a blender and blend until smooth.

- Pass the mixture through a fine mesh sieve to strain it.

- Serve over ice.

Nutritional value: Calories: 182; Fat: 0.7g; Carbohydrates: 47.6g; Fiber: 3.6g; Protein: 2.2g

3. Orange Turmeric Smoothie

Ingredients:

- 2 oranges, peeled and chopped
- 1 banana
- 1 teaspoon turmeric
- 1 teaspoon honey
- 1 cup almond milk
- Ice (optional)

Preparation:

- Combine all ingredients to a blender and blend until smooth.

- Add ice if desired, serve and enjoy immediately.

Nutritional value: Calories: 253; Fat: 3.7g; Carbohydrates: 55.1g; Fiber: 7.3g; Protein: 3.9g

4. Kale Pineapple Smoothie

Ingredients:

- 2 cups kale leaves
- 1 cup chopped pineapple
- 1 banana
- 1/2 cup coconut water
- 1/2 lemon, juiced

Preparation:

- Combine all ingredients to a blender and blend until smooth.
- Add ice if desired, serve in a glass and enjoy immediately.

Nutritional value: Calories: 275; Fat: 2.1g; Carbohydrates: 64.3g; Fiber: 8.5g; Protein: 7.5g

5.   Beet and Carrot Juice

Ingredients:

- 2 beets, peeled and chopped
- 4 carrots. peeled and chopped
- 1 apple, chopped
- 1/2 lemon, juiced

Preparation:

- Combine all ingredients to a juicer and juice.
- Serve over ice.

Nutritional value: Calories: 157; Fat: 0.6g; Carbohydrates: 38.6g; Fiber: 9.6g; Protein: 3.6g

Fighting Inflammation: How Juicing Can Help

Inflammation is a natural response of the immune system to fight off infections and injuries. However, chronic inflammation can lead to various health problems such as heart disease, diabetes, and cancer. Juicing can be an effective way to combat inflammation as it provides a concentrated dose of anti-inflammatory nutrients. Here are some recipes for anti-inflammatory juices and smoothies:

1.   Pineapple Turmeric Juice Ingredients:

Ingredients

- 1 cup pineapple chunks
- 1-inch piece of fresh turmeric
- 1/2 lemon, peeled
- 1/4 teaspoon black pepper
- 1/2 cup water

Preparation:

- Juice the pineapple, turmeric, and lemon in a juicer.

- Stir in black pepper and water.

- Serve immediately.

Nutritional Value: This juice is rich in bromelain, a compound found in pineapple that has anti-inflammatory properties. Studies have found that curcumin, an ingredient in turmeric, has the potential to reduce inflammation throughout the body.

2.   Carrot Ginger Juice Ingredients:

- 4 carrots, peeled and chopped
- 1-inch piece of fresh ginger
- 1/2 lemon, peeled
- 1/2 cup water

Preparation:

- Juice the carrots, ginger, and lemon in a juicer.

- Stir in water.

- Serve immediately.

Nutritional Value: Carrots are rich in beta-carotene, an antioxidant that helps reduce inflammation in the body. Ginger contains gingerol, a compound that has anti-inflammatory properties.

3. Green Machine Smoothie Ingredients:

Ingredients

- 1 cup kale
- 1/2 cucumber
- 1/2 green apple
- 1/4 avocado
- 1/2 lemon, peeled
- 1/2 cup water

Preparation:

- Combine and Blend all ingredients in a blender until smooth.

- Serve immediately.

Nutritional Value: Kale is a great source of vitamin C, an antioxidant that helps reduce inflammation in the body. Cucumber contains silica, a mineral that helps reduce inflammation. Avocado contains healthy fats that have anti-inflammatory properties.

4.   Beetroot and Berry Smoothie Ingredients:

Ingredients

- 1 small beetroot, peeled and chopped
- 1 cup of assorted berries consisting of strawberries, blueberries, and raspberries.
- 1/2 banana
- 1 tablespoon honey
- 1/2 cup water

Preparation:

- Combine and Blend all ingredients in a blender until smooth.
- Serve immediately.

Nutritional Value: Beetroot is rich in betaine, a compound that has anti-inflammatory properties. Berries contain anthocyanins, antioxidants that help reduce inflammation in the body. Banana contains tryptophan, an amino acid that helps reduce stress and anxiety.

5.   Golden Milk Smoothie Ingredients:

Ingredients

- 1 cup unsweetened almond milk
- 1/2 teaspoon ground turmeric
- 1/2 teaspoon ground cinnamon
- 1/2 inch piece of fresh ginger
- 1/2 teaspoon honey
- 1/2 cup ice cubes

Preparation:

- Combine and Blend all ingredients in a blender until smooth.
- Serve immediately.

Nutritional Value: Turmeric and ginger contain compounds that have anti-inflammatory properties. The consumption of cinnamon can aid in the regulation of blood sugar levels and the reduction of inflammation. Almond milk is rich in vitamin E, an antioxidant that helps reduce inflammation in the body.

CHAPTER FIVE

INCORPORATING JUICING INTO YOUR DAILY ROUTINE

HOW TO MAKE JUICING A SUSTAINABLE HABIT

Making juicing a sustainable habit can be challenging, but it is not impossible. Here are some tips to help:

1. **Set realistic goals:** Start small by incorporating juicing into your routine once a day or a few times a week. Once you become more at ease, you can raise the frequency.

2. **Make it convenient:** Keep your juicer or blender in an easily accessible place, and make sure you have a steady supply of fresh

produce. Consider prepping your ingredients ahead of time to save time.

3. **Experiment with flavors:** Don't be afraid to try new fruits and vegetables to keep things interesting. Mix and match flavors to find combinations that you enjoy.

4. **Get support:** Find a friend or family member who is also interested in juicing and make it a shared experience. Join online communities or social media groups for inspiration and support.

5. **Focus on the benefits:** Remember why you started juicing in the first place. Focus on the health benefits and how it makes you feel.

By incorporating these tips into your routine, you can make juicing a sustainable habit that supports your overall health and wellness.

Tips for Storing and Freezing Juice

Here are some tips for storing and freezing juice:

1. **Store juice in airtight containers**: When storing juice, use airtight containers to prevent air and light from degrading the quality of the juice.

2. **Use glass containers:** Glass containers are preferred over plastic containers as they don't leach chemicals into the juice and are more eco-friendly.

3. **Store juice in the refrigerator:** Store juice in the refrigerator as soon as possible after juicing to prevent bacterial growth.

4. **Freeze juice in small portions:** If you have excess juice that you can't consume within a few days, freeze it in small portions. This will make it easier to thaw and consume later.

5. **Label and date your juice**: Make sure to label and date your juice containers, so you know how long they have been stored.

6. **Freeze juice in ice cube trays**: You can also freeze the juice in ice cube trays and then transfer the cubes to a freezer bag. This allows you to easily add a few cubes to smoothies or other recipes.

7. **Thaw juice slowly:** When thawing frozen juice, do it slowly in the refrigerator or on the countertop. Avoid using a microwave, as this can heat the juice unevenly and degrade its quality.

By following these tips, you can store and freeze your juice properly and ensure that it stays fresh and tasty for longer.

Cleaning Your Juicer: Tips and Tricks

Cleaning your juicer is an important step in maintaining its longevity and ensuring that it produces high-quality juice. Here are some tips and tricks for cleaning your juicer:

1. **Disassemble the juicer:** Before cleaning, make sure to turn off and unplug the juicer. Then, disassemble the juicer into its various parts.

2. **Rinse with water:** After disassembling, rinse each part of the juicer under running water. This will remove any excess pulp or juice that may have accumulated during the juicing process.

3. **Soak in warm water:** For more thorough cleaning, soak the juicer parts in warm water mixed with a few drops of dish soap. This

will help to loosen any remaining pulp or debris.

4. **Scrub with a brush:** Use a soft-bristled brush to scrub the juicer parts gently. This will help to remove any stubborn debris or stains.

5. **Rinse and dry:** Once the parts are clean, rinse them thoroughly with water to remove any soap residue. Then, dry them completely with a clean towel before reassembling the juicer.

6. **Clean the juicer body:** Use a damp cloth to wipe down the exterior of the juicer body. Avoid using any abrasive cleaners or solvents, as these can damage the juicer's finish.

By following these tips and tricks for cleaning your juicer, you can help to ensure that it stays in good working condition and produces high-quality juice every time.

Ideas for Adding Juice to Your Meals and Snacks

Adding juice to your meals and snacks is a great way to incorporate more fruits and vegetables into your diet. Here are some ideas:

1. **Smoothie bowls:** Top a smoothie with granola, nuts, and fresh fruit for a filling and nutritious breakfast or snack.

2. **Salad dressings:** Use fresh juice as a base for a homemade salad dressing. Lemon or lime juice works well, or try using apple juice for a sweeter taste.

3. **Marinades:** Use the juice to marinate meat or tofu for added flavor and nutrition. Try

using orange juice or pineapple juice for a tropical twist.

4. **Soups:** Use fresh vegetable juice as a base for homemade soups. Carrot or tomato juice works well, or try blending kale or spinach into your soup for added nutrition.

5. **Popsicles:** Freeze your favorite juice in a popsicle mold for a healthy and refreshing summer treat.

6. **Fruit-infused water:** Add a splash of fresh juice to your water for a tasty and hydrating beverage.

7. **Cocktails:** Use fresh juice as a mixer for cocktails. Try using grapefruit juice in a margarita, or cranberry juice in a vodka tonic.

By adding juice to your meals and snacks, you can increase your daily intake of fruits and vegetables and reap the many health benefits that juicing has to offer.

CONCLUSION

In conclusion, juicing is a great way to boost your health and wellness. By incorporating fresh fruits and vegetables into your diet, you can improve your digestion, boost your immune system, fight inflammation, manage stress, and even look and feel younger. With the right tools and knowledge, juicing can become a sustainable and enjoyable habit. So why not give it a try and start reaping the numerous benefits of juicing? Remember to always choose organic produce, clean your juicer regularly, and experiment with different recipes to keep things interesting. Happy juicing!

Your Next Steps for Juicing Success

Congratulations on completing this book on juicing! You are now equipped with the knowledge and tools to start your juicing journey toward a healthier and happier you.

To ensure your success in juicing, here are some recommended next steps:

1. Choose a juicer that fits your needs and budget. Remember, the right juicer is essential for achieving optimal results.

2. Start with the basic juicing recipes provided in this book and gradually experiment with new recipes and ingredients.

3. Incorporate juicing into your daily routine. Set aside time for juicing and make it a priority in your schedule.

4. Consider joining a juicing community or group to share your experiences and get inspiration from others.

5. Keep learning about juicing and its benefits. Read books, watch videos, and attend

workshops to deepen your knowledge and stay motivated.

Remember, juicing is not just a temporary fad, but a sustainable lifestyle that can transform your health and well-being. With patience, commitment, and creativity, you can make juicing an enjoyable and rewarding habit for life. Happy juicing!

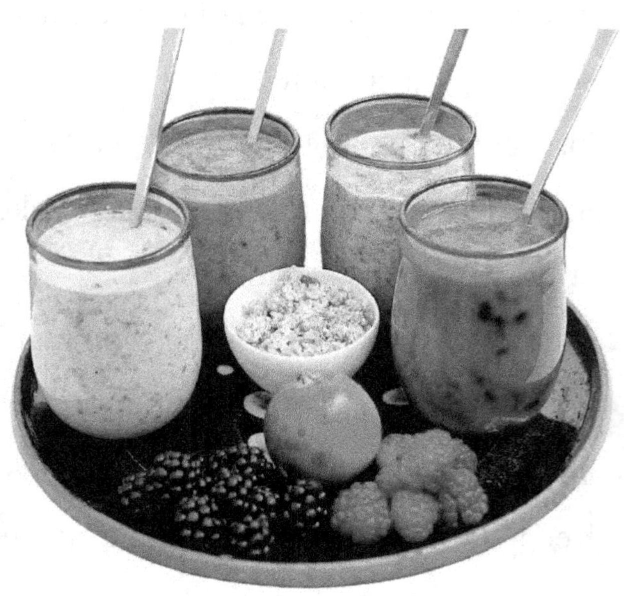

9 798386 289720